I0486162

It never seems to leave me. I mean it's just always there and do you know the thing? I can't seem to think it, say it or write it without thinking I'm being dramatic. I can't even think about it without thinking there is actually nothing wrong with me.

It started again today (12/10/2015) although in fairness I knew it was coming. I've been drinking a lot, I've been just all over the place, my temper has been short, I've been phenomenally short on patience and did I mention that I've been drinking a lot? I just don't feel like this is ever going to lift. I should be at the peak of my happiness the now, I should be king of the world, top of the world, basically any sort of happiness reference should be inserted here.

..but it's not.

I just wish I knew how to deal with this, I wish I could do something constructive rather than what feels like 'mentally menstruate', that's the best way I can describe it, I apologise about that reference but I feel it's the best one to use. It's how it feels though. At this very moment I just feel like absolute fucking shit and there's nothing I can actually do about it. That's the thing that gets me about it. If there was something I could do I would do it… but I can't.

I was sitting on the train tonight and I couldn't look straight ahead. I kept flicking between music, I kept screwing my face up, looking down, up, left right. It was like I was trying to replicate the original 'Sonic the Hedgehog' cheat using my face. (Up, Down, Left, Right, A + Start) I mean I just couldn't sit still, I think part of it was down to the fact that when I feel like this I don't want to hide any of it. I don't want to sit and look like everyone else, I don't want to play on my phone like anyone else, I don't want to look at anyone else… I am not everybody else and the sooner I realise that the better. I'm hurting just now and I could actually just sob, I could drop everything I'm doing just now and sob. I could cry my eyes out, maybe that'll make me feel better?

So I know what the general reaction to this is and I know what the thinking is going to be when I say it but I don't care, I'm going to say it anyways...

.. I need alcohol.

Yes, I know it's a depressant, yes I know it doesn't help but with me it does. I spend a lot of my time searching, I spend a great deal of my time searching actually. I don't know who I am, I'll freely admit this, I don't know where I'm going in life or what I actually want to achieve. I don't know whether to laugh or cry, if I'm seen as bold or a dumbass. I don't know what people see of me, I don't know what my parents see of me and I sure as hell don't know what I see of me. It absolutely tears me into lots of tiny pieces, I accept it though because that's the way I'm wired. I accept it and I deal with it but today.. ugh today I can't accept it because as well as pondering what my life means to me and who I am and who I want to be and the nine million other thoughts in my head I've got the super fun time of my mind racing to deal with. Happy.. fucking days. I mean happy days. So as well as having an already bursting mind I've also got the fun of my mind in warp drive mode, brilliant. Absolutely fucking top class, I could not be any happier right now. I mean... as well as managing everything else I've got going on let's add more things on to it because more always helps right?

No, not right. Wrong, fucking... wrong. It's all fucking wrong right now and I'll admit that. The question is the same as it always is.

'What's causing it'? Maybe nothing is causing it, maybe it's the fact that we're in the process of changing from season to season. Maybe it's the fact it's getting dark quicker now, maybe it's because I've been under a lot of stress the last few weeks or maybe it's down to the fact that my sheer hatred of people and my inability to work them out is coming to the surface. There, I said it. Yea', I do hate people, I have a lot of great people in my life but generally I do have a lot of hate for them. I particularly hate 'gameshow people'. You know the ones, the ones that know an answer but because they know it they'll milk the fucking cunt right out of the fucking thing. Oh god I hate that, why can't you just answer it? Why can't you just pick A,B or heaven forfend even fucking C? Why do you have to kick the arse out of it and make yourself look like a first class fucking idiot. I apologise about the language but it's going to be a recurring thing so I'm afraid you'll need to adjust. I swear a lot at the best of times, never mind when I'm mentally down and I'm ranting. So, apologies but, it's going to happen.

Do you want to know what I often think of? I often think about running away. Maybe I could, I don't think people care as much for me as they say they do. Often I feel like I'm a convenience in people's lives and I'm there when I'm needed for advice or something. Now I might be well off the mark with this but it's something that's been nagging me for the last couple of months. I just feel that maybe I'm not cut out for this 21st century living stuff; maybe I'm not cut out for social media, smartphones and civilisation. I don't think social media and me mix when I feel like this. I need to stay off it because it's at times like these everything really irritates me. The thing is though, generally everything does irritate me, I am a misanthrope. Maybe it's about time I accepted it. Maybe if I accept I hate people and stop faking interest in people I'll feel better? Maybe if I just act like myself then I'll feel better. Maybe I could do everything I should and I'll never feel better? At the moment that's what feels like the most plausible theory. So this question is going to crop up repeatedly again but once again, I guess you'll just need to adjust. 'Do you know something'? So, do you know something? I don't even know why I'm typing this up, I mean what am I actually looking to achieve out of it? I've written three before and all that it's done is given me a temporary lift. I mean all of that just for a temporary release? Great. So at least I can stop lying to myself and say that I write because it makes me feel better because it fucking doesn't and why should it? There's no reason that me tearing myself apart should make me feel better. It should do the exact opposite and it should make me question what the fuck I am doing. What the fuck am I doing?

And the answer is… I don't know. Like with ninety percent of things in my head I just don't know and that's one of the things that rankles me, it's one of those things that just eats away at me and slowly turns all the good to hate. I don't know if I need to be louder or quieter, I don't know if I talk too much or not enough. I debate my own dress sense constantly and something I've touched on previously in prior works, I analyse every single thing I say.

Maybe it is actually best if I ditch the smartphone, the social media accounts and all the chat services and just go native. Get an old phone and use it for calls & texts and that's it. Do I need to know what everyone is up to at all times and vice versa? No, probably not. Do I have the resolve and the conviction to follow through with such an idea? No, absolutely not. I come up with all of these good ideas but I never follow them through. That's a huge failing of mines, once again something I'm really honest with and happy to admit, I'm good at admitting my failings, I just need to be better at following them up. I'm crap at following them up. Actually I'm not very good at doing anything and I'm not saying this in an attempt to get people to kiss my ass and make me feel better. I'm saying it as I genuinely believe I'm actually not really good at anything. I'm an average gamer, worker, snooker player, friend. I don't really have anything I excel at, nothing I can say 'Do you know what? I'm really fucking good at this'. Well actually.. that's not true because I'm really good at these:

- Tearing myself apart
- Upsetting myself
- Over-analysing
- Over-thinking

So yea' actually I am really good at things but unfortunately nothing that's going to do anything positive for me. Ugh didn't think I could make myself feel much worse but I've just managed to do that very thing. Congratulations Dave you fucking tit. Maybe it's time to go back to the docs, maybe it's time that I just cut everyone out of what's happening, maybe it's time for me to start heading down to the basement again and start fighting all over again. I can't take this, I mean I can't… physically or mentally take this shit. I've got a work life to balance and adding this on top is like adding one too many bricks on Jenga, ugh. I just don't feel right just now, once again though I know I've not been feeling right again and it's not just because of the increase in alcohol and the mood swings, this time I've just been feeling detached from everything, this is a new thing before the depression has hit. This has been an altogether new experience and it's not necessarily a bad thing. Let me explain:

I'm pretty intense, I'm exactly what you'd expect in a Scotsman, I'm angry, fiery, a nationalist and a big drinker. I would say it's a pretty fair statement to say I never switch off and I don't. I'm always fired up, ready, alert etc. Even when I drink I find it hard to shut off because my mind is always ticking, it's always thinking of things and I'm working in tandem with it trying to analyse what it throws at me. I'm a deep, deep person, I think I hide it well in social circles & work but when I'm alone I do analyse things and think. What do I think about? Basically, the above plus nine trillion other things at any one time, it's no wonder my head is fucked. Is it fucked though? It's definitely fair to say that what I experience isn't normal but is my mind fucked? No, I don't think so. I think saying that is a dramatization and this is being written in fact, not blown up by ridiculously big exaggerations. Is that what my head does? Does it take things and just blow them out of proportion? I don't know, maybe? It comes back to that ever recurring statement though…

'I don't know'. The thing is, I don't though and it bugs me. I'm thirty-three, thirty-four in general and I feel like my life is going absolutely fucking nowhere. I'm back with my folks temporarily and I don't want to be around them and I don't want to be on my own. I never ever want to be the place where I'm at and that isn't an exaggeration that is one hundred percent fact. When I'm at work I look forward to going home, when I'm at home I look forward to going to bed, when I'm in bed I look forward to getting up, when I..

..I mean you get the idea right but I'm never comfortable in the place where I am, that slightly concerns me. I'm probably at my happiest when I'm at work because I've got tasks to focus on, my mind's got to be focused on the job in hand and that's fine. I can handle that, I like that, it's one of the few things I do like. The problems start when I'm outside of work because I'm lost, I nomad my way around my hometown, normally bouncing between pubs and writing. It's just my way and I accept that. I know this has started with a lot of swearing and vibes of I hate myself but I normally manage this pretty well, it's just the times I can't manage it the bad stuff goes down.

I'll be frank and upfront right now. I don't really know where I'm going with this and I don't know what's going to come out so you'll need to bear with me. I don't know right now what I'm thinking, well that's a lie actually because there's quite a lot going on that I conscious of. The dislike of social media is one, the (general) dislike of people is another and this is one thing that I've definitely been thinking lately, I wrote it down last week and it's something I can't seem to shake. I was in one of my local pubs in Falkirk having a pint and writing as I do. Nothing was forthcoming so I had another pint and then I checked my phone, I kept getting messages so I kept pulling my phone out and replying (as you do). It was only then I looked round and realised that I'm tied to my phone. I was pausing my writing to use my phone and since then I've been looking around and seen other people tied to their phone, tied to social media and tied to whatever app they're looking at. I wrote something interesting and something I wasn't expecting. I wrote 'I am clone 15011982'. Now 15011982 is just my birthday but I feel that I am just another insignificant member of the smartphone generation, I am a part of 'Generation Why', generation smartphone, generation app, generation anti-social and the more I think about it, the more I wretch inside. The more I hate myself for being a part of it. I hate the fact I can now sit on my phone in a social environment, use my phone and it's now considered socially acceptable.

It's not socially acceptable, it's downright fucking rude is what it is. The thing is though and I know it's going to happen is this'll pass and I'll just go back to being tied to my phone. Why should I be though? It's just not right and it doesn't sit well with me. I need to do something about it but as always I won't, I NEVER follow-up on anything. When I'm in this state I have really good ideas, I know this sounds like a contradiction but when I feel like this I do actually have some really good ideas and clear thinking. I mean granted it doesn't happen often but sometimes everything calms and I can see things the way I want to. So going back to this jotting down about me being 'clone 15011982'. Am I? Are we all just different versions of ourselves? I feel like I am, I feel I'm just average guy #3 with the build of baggy trousers with chains, a shaved head and a horseshoe moustache. Am I any different to guy #4 with his trendy clothing and in-trend hairstyle? No. We're one and the same. The only thing that differs is guy #4 has a lot trendier clothing on, less of a belly than me and probably gets more sex in one week than I do in three years. That aside are we all different? No. (Obviously this is all opinion, just more of the crap that goes on inside when I'm out having drinks.)

It's just this never ending soul-searching that mystifies me. I don't even know why I keep doing it because I don't really know what I'm searching for. Is it tranquillity? Is it stability? Is it just that little bit of sanity that staves away the demons? Once again, I don't know. It drives me absolutely fucking nuts because it goes from thinking to obsession, I can lose hours thinking and when you really break it down it's really hours thinking about absolutely fucking nothing. I mean, is this going to be me when I'm in my sixties and seventies, is there something drastic that's going to change in the next thirty-years? Am I even going to be here in two years? If you were to ask me that question could I give you an honest answer?

No, I couldn't because I actually don't know and that's one of the times where I'm quite happy to say that I don't know. Since we're there I'd be as well addressing it. Suicide is still a frequent thought in my head, it's maybe not as prominent or as strong as it was but it's still there just running in the background, I see it and I know it's still present, I deal with it, it's fine but it's something that carries relevance. It all comes back to how I feel in society and the thoughts over the last couple of months have been along the lines of wanting to exclude myself completely from social circles. Granted I've not said anything but how do you say something like that? There's no easy way to say to people, especially people I'm close to that I want nothing to do with anything anymore. That's how I feel and I think that's the first time since I started writing it's the first honest thing I've managed to dig out from inside of me, I'll say it again just so I can affirm it:

'I want nothing to do with anything anymore'.

Yip. It's true, the more I analyse it and the more I read it the more I want to do it and the more I want to do it. I don't do drama and situations well, I never have. It's one of the three thousand and sixty-five reasons I'm presently single. I just don't do drama and arguments and all that shit, I've got enough on my plate without worrying about a girlfriend who most likely will drive me up the fucking wall and vice-versa. Actually, I'm quite happy being single because not only can I do what I want when I want it also means when this strikes I can shut myself off from everyone and deal with it. Could I do that in a relationship? Hmm probably not, I think I'd find that hard. In fact scrap that, I think it'd be a nightmare so yea', happy to be single.

What is this? I mean what is causing this? Is it imbalance, is it the change in season? Stress? Change in season is plausible and I don't want to over-look the fact that this time last year is when I had my worst ever struggle with depression, that's definitely a factor I do not want to over-look. It doesn't make it any easier though, it doesn't make it easier to manage/deal with. Social media isn't helping, whilst typing this up I'm thinking about ways to disengage social media and leave my friends validated because let's face it. Why should I think of myself, I mean, there's nothing wrong with me right? It's me throwing a bit of a moody, toys out the pram right? WRONG. The sooner I start accepting that me & social media don't get on the better. I'm not built for cat updates/check-ins/baby pics and various tripe motivational quotes. If I'm being frank and honest I bore myself with social media updates so god knows what my friends & virtual friends think. The thing is though right, I'm going to do it and that's fine because I feel like total shit the now. I know I do and I've got to work through this. The good thing is I know I'll work through it and that's fine. The thing that annoys me though is when I feel better I'll want to go back on it, why though? Why do I want to go back on social media? Boredom? Obsession? OCD? I don't fucking know but I'm looking at it right now (12/10/2015) and it's just fucking shit. I can see a baby on my feed and yet another witty, funny meme shared between friends. Do you know what social media is? In-jokes, tonnes and tonnes of in-jokes intertwined between various feeds. God I actually hate it, I'm actually feeling this is therapy, you know the classic phrase 'Let it out', well this is me letting it out so here goes...

*deep breath & 1...2....3'.

This all started with something that I couldn't shake from about four, five years ago, it was when I first went through my first real battle with depression and it's stuck with me ever since. 'I was born in the right mind but born at the wrong time'. Yip, I actually agree with that and the writings I jotted down confirmed that, I looked back at them frequently and most things came back to that exact thought process. I wish I was the age I am now but in the sixties, seventies or eighties. I embrace technology but my head can't cope with the sheer amount of data and endless pointless arguments. I think too much at the best of times so when I see various postings/arguments/links/memes/baby pics/cat pics/food pics/arguments/arguments/FUCKING GOD DAMN ARGUMENTS my head just.. can't handle it, it doesn't accept it, it rejects it and quite right. Do I need to know where people are checking in, what they're up to, what their cat or pet is doing and likewise. No, the answer thankfully is a resounding, confident, over-whelming no. I check social media out of sheer boredom and for what? What is the big deal with it? I need to log out of social media and log in to what my head is actually telling me, that might be a fucking start. In fact, that IS a start.

Now I'm not trying to get across that I'm holier than thou and fucking perfect in social media, I'm not and I know I'm not but it all ties in with how I've been feeling the last few months and that links back to the whole 'I feel like a convenience', social media just helps me affirm that fact. I need a break from it, I need to come off of it or the breakdown that ensues will be epic. I'm not ready for that, there's too much on my plate just now for me to have an epic breakdown. I've got things to manage but one-hundred social media and me need to split up. Why should I constantly feel like what I've put above and continue to go on it, it does nothing for me so if I feel like I do and I'm on social media is this going to make me feel any better? No. Is it going to lift me? No. It's going to have the exact opposite effect, social media to me is what alcohol is to other people who suffer with depression and that is a depressant. If you can use it right then I guess it's great but for people that can't use it right or cope with it well, it needs to go so goodbye social media. I'm not confident but I hope I never ever see you again.

Suicide.

So, there it is. Let's just bring it right into play so there's no pussy-footing around it. It's there, it's in my head so be as well getting it down so I can look at it. So what am I seeing when I look at it?

I see nothing; I look at it as if I'd just written the word 'socks' or 'coffee', no big deal. It's a thought isn't it? This thought used to terrify me, it would cause me to cry but now it just sits there like the ten million other things and it has no effect. I keep going back to it and looking at it, yip, absolutely nothing. I don't feel good just now, I mean I think I've maybe mentioned/conveyed that over the previous pages but just in case there's any doubt, I'm not feeling good but even when I feel good suicide still floats around my head, it's just always there, sometimes in the background, sometimes right at the very back of my head and sometimes it pops in there just for no reason. The good thing, in fact the important thing is the fact that it is never ever at the front of my head. If it's at the front of my head then yea', I know things are serious. The thing that would worry anyone else with this is I think it's something that will happen someday and I hope you appreciate that I am being completely honest here. I just don't see myself getting old, I see myself committing suicide and I'm not ashamed to admit it, I think there will come a day when I've fought and fought and I just can't fight anymore. I hope I'm wrong of course but no-one knows my mind like I do and no-one knows their mind better than the person that's living inside of it. I've thought about it, analysed it, assessed it and then over-analysed it but yea', I think maybe sometime about mid-forties? It's just something I can't shake and I'm glad that I can't because I think it's healthy. Here's the reasoning:

I have been very lucky so far in life where I've not really had any tragedy, obviously I've had sadness but I've not had a totally catastrophic death that's thrown me miles off-course, I know I've still to have that but here's the thing about that, I'm prepared for it. I have to be. I cannot allow myself to be caught off-guard with a death and when I say a catastrophic death I mean a family member. I've built up my mind for it as I need to be ready for it happening, that is going to sound incredibly morbid but I need to do what's right for me. I need to prepare myself for burials/cremation, grieving and mourning and although it's not a nice subject I need to think about long-term mental health. On the flip side though, my death may come first because day-to-day I just need to evaluate this and deal with it. I still believe that it's going to be an achievement to go past thirty-five. That's still there and that's still ever present in my head, floating around there with organisation, planning for my day and suicide. These thoughts are normal, they're not normal to everyone else but they are normal to me. Considering all that goes on in my head I think I do pretty fucking well to manage my head, of course I'm going to have days like this, depression's a bitch like that. It strikes when we don't expect it, that's the nature of the beast and that's the reasons why the demons are so hard to face at times. They catch you cold. I'm lucky I generally know, I generally get a feeling so I can stick the walls up and curl up, ready to brace, face and deal with them. I don't know if that's common but do you know the thing is? I don't really care. It helps me and in times like this when I feel trapped in my own mind I have to do whatever it takes to power through the wall on the other side. It's just... it's that whole time when I'm stuck between the walls (i.e. now) that just absolutely sucks. It's just a never-ending cycle of regret, pain and being lost. It eats at me, takes chunks out of me, ruins any good thought/intention I have and most importantly/annoyingly of all it causes me just to block everyone out. The good thing is I'm learning to accept that though, as I'm getting older I'm definitely getting better at dealing with it, my mental stamina is getting better and generally people don't actually know when I'm suffering. I say generally and that's because when I'm suffering I now say to people openly. Like tonight when I came into work I got asked how I was. Honestly guys? Yea' not good and the words used were 'I know something's wrong', people respect that and I appreciate it. Tonight it's just a case of doing whatever gets me through my shift, I need that approach. My head is single-tracked tonight, the only thing I focus on is getting to seven am so I can go home and sleep.

Don't get me wrong, I know I manage this well and I don't want a picture painting misery. I take a lot of comfort in just how strong I am and for all that goes on yea', I'm fucking proud of myself and how I take hits and keep on running. The part I dread the most is being in any social environment, at times like this I need my bed, a notepad and a cup of tea. I don't care for anyone or anything else right now; my sole focus is on me, myself and I. I was on the train to work and I just didn't handle it well. I just wanted to bury my head in my hands and cry, there were so many people, there were so many people laughing, checking their phones. The only thing I could take comfort in was the fact the sun was setting and the world was pretty through my yellow shades, they've been through a lot with me and for this fight I'm going to need them again. When I have them on I feel invisible, detached, stealth. I need them actually otherwise I'd be a mess. I've had them for a year and they've seen me at my worst, they're like battle-scars and the reason I go to them is because they give me strength. They're not pretty but I don't care, as I say whatever it takes to get me through. In times like this and I know this is going to sound silly but I need them, they're necessary. They're up there with the need to be alone, my bed, my notepad and my tea. They're vital. Maybe it's best if I just cut ties with everyone, so I can truly deal with this on my own, I just can't shake this whole feeling of being a convenience in my friends lives. Once again it's something that started as a nagging thought at the back of my mind and it's been pushing its way forward ever since. Maybe that's the direction I need to go? Ugh I digress. Wanna know where I feel I'm at the now? No, well I'm going to tell you anyways. I feel like I'm in the middle of fucking nowhere, it's pitch black and I'm bang in the middle of ten million junctions, that's where I feel I am and it's somewhere I get tired of being. Maybe it would be better if I just disappeared, started again. Maybe it'd be better if I just started again, moved somewhere new and just forgot everything about everything I've ever known. Maybe it's better if I'm dead? Maybe that'll finally quench the burning deep inside my soul. I mean what the fuck is it going to take? Keep bearing my soul every four or five months for temporary release? Is that what I'm striving for, is that what my release is? That's my crumb of comfort? Wow well fucking sign me up and hold me back. Anything has to be better than this; anything has to be better than feigning interest in things and people. Feigning interest in stories and fake laughing, acting like I care, acting like I give a fuck when really I don't. I genuinely don't give a fuck but rather than me following my convictions I talk myself out of it. This is making me sound ungrateful to everyone that's stood by me, it's not. I am grateful. In fact who am I even talking to, none of my 'friends' are going to read this! Haha that's amazing! It's taken me over five thousand words to realise that I'm ranting against myself, fucking brilliant Dave you first class cunt. Honest to fuck see whatever the opposite of The Turner Prize is you would definitely be in the running for it.

I need some time away from people, the way this is going this isn't going to end well. As I'm typing this my hatred is growing but I look calm. I am calm I just…. I just get annoyed by too much, I get annoyed by commentators saying obvious statements, I get annoyed by people stating the obvious, like weather forecasters pointing out at this point in time (12/10/2015) that it's getting colder in the UK and Australia are seeing temperatures up to twenty-nine degrees fahrenheit. Well… obviously, we're coming into winter and they're edging towards summer so yea', there is a chance that our weather is going to get colder and theirs is going to get warmer. It's like when I'm watching golf and they interview the guy or girl that's one and the first question they ask is 'How do you feel'? How do you think they feel you fucking dumbass, they've just WON the very event they've just entered. You don't walk up to someone after a funeral and ask them how they're feeling so why the fuck are you asking someone that's just won something how they feel. You fucking fuckturd. See? That stuff drives me up the fucking wall.

I HATE idiocy and stupidity, definitely two of my pet peeves, once again why being a part of 'Generation Fucking Why' grinds my gears. It's way too accessible for people to be idiots and stupid. You just need to log on to our good friend social media to see why. I'm going to go back so bear with me again but there is a point and I'll start with four words..

'The Scottish Independence Referendum'.

This... drove... me... nuts. Now before I start I'd like to point out I am a proud Scot and I voted Yes BUT I didn't do it blindly, I sat and deliberated for months about it, I wanted to vote Yes but only if I thought it was sustainable and the right thing for our wee country. Anyway I voted Yes and we somehow voted No, I'm not getting into politics because I need to feel better, not worse.

Social media was an absolute fucking nightmare and I mean from July until the actual voting day it was chaos, I didn't know so many idiots existed, the arguments ranged from oil to culture even to personal differences! I mean it was fucking nuts and I hated being part of it. People fell out, harsh words were exchanged, digital friendships were thrown away and of course people of two certain big football clubs in Scotland had their usual unique, well thought out inputs. My point is this, everyone is entitled to an opinion, that's granted but what my head can't process is people throwing completely illogical arguments about, people that make really stupid points or the worst, people that actually don't know what the fuck they're talking about. I loved the independence referendum, I genuinely enjoyed watching the televised debates, I like debates as long as they remain somewhat factual. People who have access to social media have a free reign to do what they want and it's just a shame that a really good chance for lively debate turned into a mud-slinging match with digital ramifications. Anyway, we voted no and that's the end of it. Enough on it because it's starting to boil my blood, moving swiftly on.

On the plus side it at least pulled me away from my head for a wee bit and to be honest I feel a wee bit better for it, whether I'll feel better at seven o'clock tomorrow morning is a different story.It just irritates me, I just don't know if I want to be facing this the rest of my life, I mean, suicide is the last option for so many reasons but will it actually quell my pain? I've attempted it once but I tapped out. I had the balls to do it and I should have seen it through, that statement is deliberate. If I'm going to do something like that then it's not fair to have so many people suffer. If it ever comes to it again, there is no tapping out, let's get that fucking clear. If the day comes where my reasons for dying outweigh my reasons for living then I need to involve no-one. That statement should be sending chills down my spine but it doesn't. It's like the word suicide it just.. sits there, as if I'm reading a junk email, it just does absolutely nothing. Maybe I'm more ill than I thought? Well there's nothing I can do about it tonight so it'll just have to sit there. I'm a mess mentally, I don't actually know if I'm coming or going, I don't know if I want to live or die and I don't know if I want to beat this or I want this to beat me. Once again, all sounds very dramatic but this is what's going on. I got a tattoo about a month ago, actually I got two. I got a semi-colon tattooed on my neck to symbolise like the sentence, the fight isn't over and a chest piece that reads 'The Devil & God Rage inside me'. Well, they do basically because I'm always caught between good and evil basically. It's where I constantly seem to be stuck between.

I mean. Is it worth me looking at me getting help for something I may not actually want to get help on? I'm not sure. Sure I can go to the docs and bounce ideas off of him. Sure I can make these grand ideas up and I can formulate plans to deal with it but ultimately this is inside of me and it doesn't appear to be getting better. Maybe I don't want it to get better? Maybe me writing this is going to allow me to be honest and say 'I don't want to beat it'. Maybe… The more I read that back the more I can't decipher, I don't actually know if I want to or if I have the desire to do so. I feel inferior to people, I just don't feel I have anything to offer society, whether that's to do with how I feel just now or whether that's long-term I don't know. I mean that thought has been there for a while so that's definitely one I'm debating. I'm sitting just... thinking. I'm just sitting, scratching thoughts against the wall, desperately hoping one sticks there, endlessly looking down avenues for that one breakthrough that'll free me from this, that one thought or mantra that will relieve me of all this weight that's pushing my head down. I've got to. I have to. I NEED... to. If I don't do that then what chance do I have? I'm beginning to feel like this is hopeless, it's maybe not but all I can think of is removing myself from society, removing myself from friends and just leaving family and even then not letting them in. I want to run. Fight or flight is causing my hands to run cold, the blood is going to the legs prepping me to sprint away. Is that the answer? Cutting ties and just disappearing? It's definitely in there and it's stronger than suicide or any other thought I have. Do I plan it or just do it? How do I go about it? I mean I can actually feel the weight pushing my head down, my shoulders actually ache, weirdly the right one aches more than the left one but right on top of my head it feels like a weight is pushing it down, the back of my eyes hurt and my chest actually feels heavy. There's got to be something that causes this, I can't just be 'imbalanced', it's got to be more than chemical, there's something that causes this I'm sure of it. Yes I get warning signs, yes I'm grateful for them but what I'm not grateful for is how much this throws me, I'm beginning to think that there's no hope. I'm beginning to wonder if people can forgive me. Forgive me for what I don't fucking know but if it comes to it.. would they forgive me?

And here we are, back at those three fucking words..

I...

DON'T...

KNOW......

...and I don't, that's the thing. I've volunteered for a local mentalhealth charity where I stay, I done that on Wednesday of last week (07/10/2015) and I'll be honest I'm nervous. Can I handle that? Could I do it? I mean writing isn't doing it and apparently writing is very cathartic, well I'm sorry to say but it's not been fucking cathartic for me. I continually slice myself open only for the scars to heal and then bleed when it fucking well likes.

Uch the more I'm writing the worse I'm feeling, it's like I'm pulling at this wound and nothing's there, it's phantom, it feels like it's there but it's not. But I feel pain so surely where pain is there has to be something there? I mean that's not far-fetched thinking is it? That's logic? Surely? Can someone please help me, I'm floundering, grasping at straws looking for anything that's going to see me through this. I need to get through this. Maybe if I go on social media........ Aye, right who am I kidding, that'll make me feel better. I'd rather stick my head in a shredder than go back to that. My thoughts are all clashing against each other now, they're all trying to run through the same door and they're clashing, they're blocking everything so now I'm sitting trying to get some peace of mind and I'm getting static. There's nothing, there's no respite available. I'm in the worst place possible now and that's where my thoughts are racing and crashing against one another. It renders me useless, helpless and in safe mode. My mind is now entering the stage where I can't function unless the action ahead meets very strict parameters, this is the part of the depression I hate the most because I have nowhere to go, no shelter it's just like touching a raw nerve or an electric fence with the voltage full. Nothing works, nothing gives me that relief and it fucking sucks. Let me be clear, depression is a first class cunt to deal with, I don't use that word often and I am aware I've used it in this writing but it's not a word I throw about when talking about depression but I'm beginning to feel like I'm never going to beat this. It keeps coming back to that train of thought and it'll always come back to that. I'm sick of this whole thing, I know that's fairly generic but it's true. I do hate it. I hate the fact I'm now looking at the possibility of ostracizing people just to appease myself. It makes me sad.

I don't ask for much, I'm a casual gamer, I like playing snooker, I like basically hanging out with people but will I ever beat this? One of those questions that makes me feel like I'm a pre-teen that's just broken up with his 'childhood sweetheart. Do you know what fuck that? Why should I constantly feel like I'm the one that's wrong and doing things wrong? I'm not doing things wrong, I'm doing things RIGHT and I STILL FEEL AS IF I'M FUCKING WRONG. How is that possible? I'm not doing anything wrong, even at one of my lowest ebbs I'm still refusing to acknowledge that I'm not choosing this, I am not choosing to feel this way and I am most certainly not looking at suicide for the sheer fucking fun of it, let me be clear on that in case it wasn't. This is hard, this is very fucking hard, I'm bleeding my guts out here and I'm the one that feels wrong? Why? Why the fuck why??? That's not fair. That's not fair on me. This is serious fucking shit, this unhinges me and takes me away from those I love, those that stand by me and fight with me. I know I keep going over this but why in the time that I need people do I feel that this is some big weakness? It's not. It's perfectly acceptable, it's how I've trained my mind over the last nine months, ever since I attempted suicide in December last year it's what I said I would do and I've fucking done it. I've blew this open, I've written about it, I've been open about it and I've fucking dealt with it. I am dealing with it, this isn't fair. This is an affliction, a disability, a disease but here I am working through it, no-one knows I feel this way so I just.. sit in silence? Is that the way I go about it? Aye because if I do that it's going to end well isn't it? I have made such an effort to blow this open and here I am belittling myself for it. Way to go Dave, that's really healthy doing that. I don't even know what I want now, (ha! As if I did before!) I don't know what my plan of attack is, where I'm going to go and how I'm going to fucking well deal with this. (I am trying to clean up the language but I'm emotive, what can I say. I am trying though….)

I'm sitting here, it's just turned midnight and what am I doing? Trying to think, I just will not switch off. I drive myself crazy and the thing is I think I need to. I think I need to drive myself crazy. Bizarre statement? Well no not really. I like to think that by going through this it drags up a lot of the crap, kinda similar to a car running really low on petrol so it brings all the dregs of the tank up. Whereas that's not good for the car it's good for my head, I need this every once in a while but that's not to say I like it any better. I don't, I fucking hate it. I fucking hate everything right now and once again my conversations have hit a wall on social media, I swear to god I could scream just now. I don't mind conversations breaking down but three lines in I just don't get it. Am I that boring? Am I that un-interesting? Maybe I should get a tattoo across the front of my head that says 'Regular'. Would that help everyone? Would maybe fucking help me to accept that I'm just not that interesting, well according to the digital world anyways. So if the above is correct I'm writing this for the sake of my sanity. Well, maybe that's not a bad thing, it's the one thing I feel that makes sense and it's the one thing I'm barely clinging on to. Let's be honest if I don't have my sanity this thing is over, I mean if the sanity goes everything goes with it so saving that is definitely worth fighting for. At the moment though it feels about all that I can fight for?

It's tough. It's hard to accept that I am this way, I keep hoping that one day this'll dissipate and I'll get myself back permanently. It feels just now I am a chameleon version of myself, depending on what social circle I'm in adapting to the needs and character of that group. That just tells me that I need to do one of two things, I either need to:

- Be myself (*sniggers*, yea' right)
- Gradually move away from my social circles.

Option two is definitely more plausible than option one, I find it very very hard to be myself unless I'm on my own. If I'm around any single one of my friends I adapt myself to their character needs. I dare not speak my own mind, I stick to a certain formula that caters to said friend. That's horrifying, I'm reading that back and I actually do that, ugh it makes me sick that I actually do that. I need a lot of time myself, I need a LOT of time to myself, mainly because people drive me crazy, I may have mentioned that once or twice? The main reason I need a lot of time to myself is I need to process all that goes on, process, manage and then deal with it. Maybe I should spend more time on my own? Maybe that's the answer? Maybe I should just deal with whatever comes into my head on my own instead of letting it manifest itself and poison my view of others. If I don't have the others then the worst I can do is poison myself and let's face it, considering how hard this hits it wouldn't damage me that much. This is ridiculous, I mean this whole fucking thing is ridiculous. I just don't get me, I don't understand all of this. I get it but I don't fucking understand it. Maybe it's just a case of letting things take their course, managing this and seeing where it takes me. Previous works I've gotten out what's bothering me, backstories, planning and even swearing on celibacy. Aye that lasted long. See? I make these grand fucking plans and within a week or a month I'm breaking them. Do you know the best thing to do? See any plan that I say I'm going to do, ignore it because it's all just a pile of absolute fucking pish. I have the greatest of intentions but the worst will. See if I really wanted to and I mean REALLY wanted to I could give up alcohol but… I won't. Whatever I say I'm going to do is all spur of the moment, it's all fiction, and basically it's all fucking tosh. I wouldn't say I give up because that's dramatic but I am at a total loss as to who I am. I've completely lost my identity and I have completely lost my way. I'm lost, I am hopelessly lost in my life and I don't know where to go, who to turn to or what my next move is. I'm back sitting at the road with one million junctions, it's pitch black and I'm blindfolded, I have no clue what's the first step to take, what direction I'm going in or what direction I want to take. I can make the simplest thing complex, pretty ironic for a guy that prides himself on wanting the simple things. The weird thing about this whole fucking stramash is that it speaks to me about how I need a direction in life, that much I get and I appreciate it but what it doesn't do is tell me why the fuck I'm feeling like this, why am I stuck between happiness & suicide, thunder & sunshine, chalk & cheese, any sort of opposite combination you want to stick in here then stick it in. What does it matter? What does any of this matter? It won't go away, I don't know if I want it to go away, I don't know what to do and I don't know if I'll ever know what I want to do. I may be contemplating this in thirty years, I may be dead within two years. Do you know what?

I…. just.. don't know.

Just how much am I expected to bleed before the wound heals? How much further do I have to run before I can stop? Just how many walls am I going to have to blitz through before I can relax? I'm thinking back to this time last year. This time last year was by far the worst time I've ever had, I'd say that's fair considering all I went through. I went on a course of anti-depressants (which done nothing) and I stayed with my brother. He went to work and I was in the house, I didn't wash my face for forty-four days, I fought with myself day in and day out for months, I spent a lot of my time in silence staring out into nothing, I spent my days wandering from room-to-room, not doing anything, aimlessly killing time until bedtime so I could sleep, at least when I slept nothing could hurt me. I spent the best part of four months wondering if I was ever going to be myself again, I spent four long, hard months trapped between being on my own and leaving the house. Did any of my so called friends come to see me? Did they fuck, the people that told me that 'if I ever needed a chat' that they'd be there for me. The people that wished me well and said that 'a catch-up soon would be nice' didn't bother their arse. I made the effort, I went out once in Glasgow in November but it was me that made the effort, I dragged myself up and out, I put myself in a place where I hadn't been in a while, I put myself right smack bang around people, I put myself in Glasgow where there were a lot of people, not once did I feel comfortable but it was up to me to make the effort. I guess I just wasn't that important after all, I guess some people are just so full of shit that they say what you want to hear and then just forget all about you. I spent four of the longest months searching for something to grab on to and the only thing that I really ended up grabbing onto was an alcohol addiction and a desire to commit suicide. That's what my four months got me, that was the sum total of my time. I have never felt so confused, I've never had that much time to myself and I've never hated myself that much. That tearing between being on my own and going down to see my folks, the debating, the staring out the window, the wandering. The doubt, fear and self-loathing I endured was nothing short of torture, quite frankly I'm not sure how I managed four months. Ok so eventually I tried to tap out and quit, no wonder. By the end of things I was nothing but an alcoholic, alcohol had lost it's flavour as I got hammered every night. If it wasn't for my true friends & my family I wouldn't be here. That's why I fight, that's why when this gets me down I remind myself of just how much I have fought to get back up to where I am today. Yes this is a bad period but I've had worse, I've had sustained periods where I have been held prisoner in my own mind. This? This is nothing compared to what I went through but it doesn't make it any easier.

I'm writing this for a reason, there is a point to this self-mutilation. If I lay everything out there it means I can't hide, I can't hide away from it and I can't run away from it. By being honest about suicide it means I'm one step closer to finding a way to deal with this and maybe that one step is one of ten thousand, it doesn't matter. Any step I and anyone that suffers from a mental health issue can take towards being a better person I'll take, I don't care if that one step is over broken glass whilst bare-footed I'll take it. Hell I'll crawl if it means collectively we can fight through this. With mental health issues like depression just making it through a day is an achievement, by me making it through to seven am and getting to bed is an achievement. If by helping people I've got to slice myself open I'll do it. I can do it and I'm used to doing it. I bleed every day and I'm not afraid to show that. I'm a good man with a lot to give but the question I constantly ask is...

Will I get the time to give back and I think it's only fair to answer it with this...

I don't know.

I need to do something but what? Will volunteering to help people that struggle with mental health give me what I need to release myself from this or am I destined to never be freed from this. Am I going to spend the rest of my life searching for something that maybe just.. isn't there? This much is for sure, my journey hasn't been an easy one but one of the things giving me comfort is I'm still going, I'm still fighting and I'm still maintaining hope that someday I can one day break through these walls and leave them all broken behind me. Maybe one day this'll all make sense and I can manage it effectively. Maybe one day I can accept myself for who I am. My life has fantastic people in it and I am so grateful to have them in it but do I want them knowing I suffer? Well, yes if I'm suffering then they need to know, the mistake I made last year was not doing that. They thought I was fine and I wasn't, I mean I REALLY wasn't. Would I say I'm fine just now? Well, no of course I'm not because of what's been written but if it comes time to ask for help, I'll do it. Make no mistake, if I'm going to bow out I want to do it after I have explored every single option, my folks raised no quitter, I am not a quitter, I'm a scrapper and a fighter. By bleeding myself out I'm proving that I'm strong, by ripping my wounds wide open for everyone to see shows that I'm fighting. I am fighting, we're all fighting this and hopefully we can beat this. I want to keep writing things like this because it shows there is still fight left within me. If I'm not doing anything then I've given up and the story is finished, my journey has ended. I don't want my journey to end just yet, I'm not ready but for any reason if it does I need to have it cleared up that I fought, I fought with every bit of my heart, body and soul. I am fighting with heart, body and soul.

This may not make a lot of sense to people that don't suffer from mental health issues but believe me, that statement shows there's still fight in the tank, there's still a fight going on and there's commitment. It shows that although I've acknowledged that suicide doesn't scare me it's not an option I'm going to turn to easily, it's not something I'm going to turn to without taking every single step I can to beat this. I do want to beat this but...

... it's just so draining sometimes. To be honest I am still contemplating going this alone. I got burned badly last year by people whom I thought were my friends, that took a lot of getting over and that's only something that I've recently managed to deal with, attempting suicide took one month to get over, being burned by people that I thought were there for me has taken a long time to heal. I value friends and I mean I value FRIENDS, true friends. The kind of friends that stepped up last year when they knew I was miles off, the type of friends that brought me back from the edge of a balcony, friends that are there for me in the good times and also are there for me during the bad times. I worship these people, I need these people and I love these people but after last year and what I'm feeling now, is it maybe time for me to go this alone? I feel..

...I feel a sense of overwhelming detachment from them and I just don't feel the same. I will never forget what they done but things are changing inside my mind, I feel I've lost my connection with them so I think I've got a decision to make. I love them so much and I mean that, that's why I think I need to step away from them, I'm no longer the same to them, I feel it. I've tried to re-connect but let's face it, there comes a point in your life where you look at something and you're like... nope. I think that's where I am now, I've ran as far as I can with my friends and now it's time for me to deal with this on my own whatever that means. The hardest part of this is going to be having the conversations with them. I'm sure I'll miss the good times they share but also it makes sense for me to make this decision. I need to face this on my own, I need to deal with this on my own and eventually a road will open, the darkness will lift and I'll take whatever path shines brightest. Which one that'll be...

Well..

I don't know.

www.ingramcontent.com/pod-product-compliance
Lightning Source LLC
Chambersburg PA
CBHW070802180526
45168CB00004B/1717

* 9 7 8 1 5 1 7 7 9 9 7 2 4 *